Common Sense Germs

by Faye McCrae Athey

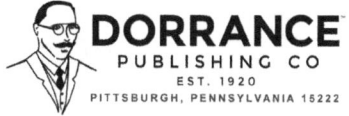

The contents of this work, including, but not limited to, the accuracy of events, people, and places depicted; opinions expressed; permission to use previously published materials included; and any advice given or actions advocated are solely the responsibility of the author, who assumes all liability for said work and indemnifies the publisher against any claims stemming from publication of the work.

All Rights Reserved
Copyright © 2014 by Faye McCrae Athey

No part of this book may be reproduced or transmitted, downloaded, distributed, reverse engineered, or stored in or introduced into any information storage and retrieval system, in any form or by any means, including photocopying and recording, whether electronic or mechanical, now known or hereinafter invented without permission in writing from the publisher.

Dorrance Publishing Co
701 Smithfield Street
Pittsburgh, PA 15222
Visit our website at *www.dorrancebookstore.com*

ISBN: 978-1-4809-1150-5
eISBN: 978-1-4809-1472-8

DEDICATION

In loving memory of Rosa Athey, Annie and James McCrae.

My goal is to bring awareness to the public. Germs are virtually everywhere, even in the rarest of places, but through *Common-*Sense *Germs,* people can begin to pay closer attention to their environment and decrease the spread of germs. I have an even greater passion for the people of GOD, and I would like to acknowledge Outreach Ministry of Sandy Hook, VA; Bishop Gilbert C. Athey, Sr.

Special thanks to Amanda Harris for all of your help and support through this process. Thank you for your inspiration Kenneth, Dominic and Tavaris McCrae; Alice Bethea, Cleola Parnell, Andrea Thomas, Pastor Frank B. Reeves, Marian B. Reeves, Nelson B. Athey and Lashelle Mallory-Athey.

BACK TO THE BASICS

Let's take a moment to think about "the beginning of time." GOD created all things, animals, human beings, plants, etc. Everything he created he said was good; it's we as humans who tend to not follow the basics and change the dynamics of things, resulting in a world of disarray. I firmly believe that God's intention for his people was for us to live a harmonious life of peace and equality, but instead, because of disobedience, we live in a world of catastrophe, violence, war, and pestilence, a world full of GERMS.

As I think about the world and how full of germs it truly is, I wonder, how did this all come to be? How are germs being spread, and how can we stop or slow down the spread of germs? Most people think about germs being spread from one person, place, or object to another, but let's factor in animals. We have regulations in place that require that we as Americans receive immunizations, but what about animals? Some travel coast to coast. Think about what type of germs or disease they might be transporting. Are we going to stop each bird in the sky and give them a flu shot? Of course not! My point is that we should not just look at humans or objects and think this is the only way germs can be spread.

There are wild animals that tend to migrate to our backyards, rummaging through our garbage, eating whatever they may find. What happens when one of these animals comes across something that may be contaminated with blood or some other bodily fluid? Although they are animals, let's not count out the possibility that they could then become the carrier of diseases and germs that we have, which can lead to a larger coverage area for the spread of germs.

I believe that if we begin to pray, avail ourselves to GOD, and use our common sense, we will witness a change in the world, one being a decrease in the spread of germs from one person or place to another.

CONTENTS

INTRODUCTION ix
CHAPTER 1: BABIES 1
CHAPTER 2: BARBERS 2
CHAPTER 3: BARS AND CLUBS 4
CHAPTER 4: BATHROOMS 5
CHAPTER 5: BEAUTY STORES 6
CHAPTER 6: CLOTHING 7
CHAPTER 7: FAST FOOD 8
CHAPTER 8: CONVENIENT STORES 9
CHAPTER 9: GROCERY AND DEPARTMENT STORES 10
CHAPTER 10: HOUSEKEEPERS 12
CHAPTER 11: MAIL 13
CHAPTER 12: MALLS 14
CHAPTER 13: MONEY 15
CHAPTER 14: NAIL SALONS 16
CHAPTER 15: OFFICE 17
CHAPTER 16: RESTAURANTS 18
CHAPTER 17: SHOES 20
CHAPTER 18: SHOE SHOPPERS 21
CHAPTER 19: LAUNDROMAT 22
CHAPTER 20: EXPECTANT MOTHERS 23
CHAPTER 21: TIPS AND TECHNIQUES 24

INTRODUCTION

The bible says, "My people perish for lack of knowledge" (Hosea 4:6 (KJV)). Society, it's time to wake up, take things back to the basics, and use our common sense. This book provides the information necessary to decrease the spread of germs, but it's up to you to practice what you learn. If you don't know, now you know!

Think about a germ as a puddle of water that you've stepped in. Quite naturally you're going to track that water wherever you walk. Germs are the same way as that puddle in some instances; they hitch a ride with their host, thus being transferred from one place to the other. How many times in a week or month do you visit your local grocery store? Have you ever thought about how many hands have touched the canned goods you're holding, or what about that loaf of bread or quart of milk? How long did it sit in the warehouse before reaching the shelves? How often are you wiping down the items you purchased from the grocery store before placing them in your cabinets or refrigerator at home? If your answer to the last question was never, then guess what? You have just contaminated your home with germs, which tend to grow in dark, cool places. All of this information is common sense. If you don't know, now you know!

As humans, we tend to get sick often, and there are simple steps we can follow to prevent this. We just need to use our common sense. I always thought I practiced good techniques, but one day, as I began to observe people in the community, I noticed proper hand techniques were not being practiced. For example, most people wash their hands after they use the bathroom, but wouldn't it make common sense to wash your hands before you use the bathroom as well? Take a moment to think about the multitude of germs that are on your hands from touching door knobs, keys, phones, etc., and you've just touched the toilet paper that you're going to use to wipe your private areas. It's common sense to wash your hands before and after you use the bathroom. Improper hand washing techniques can lead to serious illnesses.

BABIES

Most parents hate to see their innocent bundles of joy sick and would do anything to see them feel well again. We can start this process by avoiding the things that help our babies get sick: germs. We as parents need to use our common sense and accept responsibility that we are the first line of defense against our babies coming into contact with unwanted germs. Parents, we can start by simply washing our hands. How many parents change their babies without washing their hands before and afterwards? Then we reach into the diaper bag without realizing it, contaminating everything else. Also, how often do you wipe down or clean items before you place them in your diaper bag? You should remove items such as diapers from their original packing and place them in a closed, sealed container before placing it into the diaper bag. Cans of milk should always be wiped off as well. Parents, please avoid washing your babies' clothing along with yours; this is not a time that you should be attempting to conserve water. As parents, we're typically busy, but taking a few minutes to wash your hands before and after diaper changes or cleaning items before they go into your diaper bag can make the difference between a healthy baby or a sick baby.

BARBERS

If you have ever visited a barber shop, the following routine may sound familiar. You're in the barber's chair, waiting to get your hair cut, edges rounded up, or a demolition on some of that irritating ear and nose hair, and definitely a trim of the mustache or beard. These are typical things that most individuals get done when visiting the barber shop. Do you ever think about the person who was in front of you who had the same thing done? Was there any sanitation done in between clients? Imagine all of the skin contact your barber's hands, clippers, combs, etc., have encountered throughout the course of the day before they are cleaned. Clippers and razors are commonly used in barber shops, and clients are almost certain to get a cut or two during a shape-up, resulting in a possible transference of blood. How is your barber handling the sanitation of their clippers/razors in cases such as this? How often is your barber sanitizing his chair or sweeping around it? Think about lint and how it attaches to your clothing. Well, imagine all of those prior clients who sat in that barber's chair, and now some portions of their hair are possibly stuck to you. Barbers need to wash their hands before and after each client, as well as sanitize their chairs and equipment in between clients.

Companies have policies and procedures in place that dictate how their company is run and protecting the company and their employees in the event of a lawsuit. There are entities that can dictate and oversee the regulations of different types of businesses, but few are in place that ensure the safety of the public from the spread of germs—hair salons being one of these types of businesses.

Generally, as a customer in a salon, after the greetings are done, you're seated in a chair, where the stylist proceeds to prep your hair for whatever treatment you request. From the time you enter the salon till you've sat in the stylist's chair, more than likely no hand washing has been performed. The stylist then uses combs, products, etc., that have been used on other clients without any prior cleaning. This touching-and-reusing process can be harmful, spreading germs from one person to the next. The sit-under dryer tends to be one of the most overlooked apparatuses in the salon to be cleaned. Stylists need to review their procedures, then create polices that will help protect their clients, such as cleaning combs and dryers between clients, not reusing products that have been previously used on other clients.

IF YOU DIDN'T KNOW, NOW YOU KNOW!

BARS AND CLUBS

Most people who go out to bars or clubs are there to socialize, have fun, and enjoy the entertainment. Occasionally, someone may have too many drinks and get sick, throwing up on the chair, floor, table, and anything else surrounding that area. Usually there is a quick cleanup of the area and back to business as usual. Suppose you were the lucky person who got to sit in that area where the last patron just finished puking their brains out. Now you're possibly contaminated with their body fluids. Do you know their health history or what type of diseases, germs, and bacteria you may be exposed to? Imagine different people repeatedly being sick in that same area. A quick cleanup done each time—boy, that's a lot of contamination!

BATHROOM

Women, I know we have been taught to wipe front to back, but what I don't understand is why anyone would take urine from the front and put it on the back. It's common sense. What if you had a urinary tract infection, were on your menstrual, or had some other foreign drainage of some sort? How simple would it be to wipe the front, roll off some more toilet paper, and then wipe the back instead of doing it all in one sweep?

BEAUTY STORES

You must use your common sense when going into hair stores. People tend to touch, open containers, and try out the products before buying them. Usually these types of stores supply wig caps for sale to those seeking to try on a wig before purchasing it, but what about the stores that do not offer these caps? The next time you're in your local beauty store, stop and look around at the employees and customers. Check out their habits and see how easily germs can be spread.

IF YOU DON'T KNOW, NOW YOU KNOW!

CLOTHING

People often say, "I can wear this again; it's clean. I only wore it to the doctor's office and the store." Think about the doctor's office. Imagine how many sick people are going there for a checkup and sitting in the same chairs where everyone else sits. I've witnessed people go to the hospital and the very next day, they're wearing the same clothes, stating that it was clean. There is no difference between the doctor's office, hospital, etc. Your clothes should be changed daily. For example, think about the different types of professionals who may change their clothes as soon as they get home: doctors, nurses, construction workers, delivery drivers, dentists, and so forth. These individuals are using their common sense; they're either in the community or working with people from within the community all day, attracting and coming into contact with all types of germs. Why would you want to wear those same clothes for another day? Germs are virtually invisible to the naked eye. Once they've attached to your clothing, it is easier to penetrate open skin, compromising your health. It makes common sense to not wear the same clothing more than once without washing it first.

FAST FOOD

These are great places to grab a bite to eat, but it's common sense to pay close attention to how your food is being prepared and served. Typically, a cashier is up front taking orders, which requires taking money from customers' hands, and of course we don't know where they've been. By this time, a red light should be going off, saying, "Germ alert."

True story: One morning on my way to work, I stopped by a fast food restaurant to have breakfast. I ordered oatmeal and as I stood in line awaiting my order, I observed the same cashier take another order, then stop to place hot water into a cup, along with the oatmeal and fruit, before handing it to me. I immediately thought, *what is wrong with this picture?* Not once did this cashier stop to wash her hands in between touching the register, the customer's hands, handling their money, and preparing food. The spread of countless germs was passed in every action. Imagine how busy these establishments get; often you will see the cashier performing three to four different duties between customers without washing their hands, changing their gloves, or even using a hand sanitizer.

I have an even greater issue with the ketchup being placed in my food bag along with my exposed food. These packets are touched by countless hands and like most things, they had to be shipped to the restaurant, unpacked, and stored in mini-bins, allowing for a great deal of germs to come into contact with the packets. The same holds true for the napkins, straws, and utensils that are not in plastic. Your items should be individually wrapped.

CONVENIENCE STORES

Most convenient stores are like revolving doors; customers are in and out all day long, using the gas pumps, picking up snacks and food, etc. Think about the countless number of people who stop at these places and the countless amounts of germs each person may be carrying. Usually people are filling up their cars at these stores, but think about how many other people have filled up before you, which means they had to touch that same pump. Nowadays, most places have hand sanitizer by the pumps, but it is hardly a replacement for washing your hands. At some point before or after pumping gas, the cashier has to be paid, which requires touching money or your debit/credit card, which leads to the spread of more germs if your hands have not been washed.

Many of these stores have areas where food can be purchased. How often do you see customers pump their gas, pick up food, pay for items, and are off to their vehicle to eat without giving any thought to washing their hands?

GROCERY AND DEPARTMENT STORES

I consider the grocery store to be a "hands-on" place. What I mean is that most people go there to shop, and of course they are touching items as they shop. I'm almost certain that most people do not think about how many hands have touched the same canned goods they are touching or how they were stored in the warehouse prior to arriving at the grocery store. At best, the FDA ensures that food products are safe for consumption before they are sold in stores, but my concern is that there are no regulations or training on how to ensure that customers are safe when shopping at their local grocery store, department store, etc.

For example, I frequently visit the grocery store and as I'm standing in line with about eight people in front of me, I notice the cashier has on gloves, and there is nothing wrong with that. But my concern is that she is touching the cash register, customers' money, debit/credit cards, and groceries without changing gloves in between transactions. Obviously this cashier was aware of what germs are to some degree, and I commend her for attempting to protect herself from attaining germs. But look at how many others she has put at risk for the spread of germs. Imagine how many germs had collected on those pair of gloves.

Have you ever been shopping and were drawn to a table or booth with free food samples of different products? Well, most of us have. How many of you washed your hands before eating that sample, and did you think about how many others in front of you also touched that sample tray without washing their hands? Let's not even begin to talk about the fresh fruit such as grapes that so many shoppers occasionally tend to eat while pushing their shopping carts, never once washing their hands or the grapes. I enjoy eating a bag of potato chips or a candy bar, but simple items such as these can host germs from the multitude of hands that have touched them; therefore, I make sure I wipe off all of my items before I eat them.

Here are some common tips for shoppers: Always wipe your purchased items before storing them in your refrigerator or cabinets. Germs tend to grow in cold, dark places. Make sure you throw away boxes or containers that your items came in, as they could be holding bugs, mites, germs, etc. Always wipe/clean your debit/credit cards before placing them back in your wallet or purse. Think about how many transactions you've used your debit/credit card for and how many hands have touched it. If stores have antibacterial wipes for their shopping carts, why wouldn't you think everything else in the store didn't need to be wiped down as well?

Most people try on clothes before they purchase them, but think about how many other people have tried on those same items. You have no idea of their background, if they showered that day, or if they have some sort of skin infection or bacteria. You should avoid wearing or using anything before washing it, such as towels, washcloths, underwear, etc. Items such as these are usually lying on shelves, and shoppers like to touch and feel the material. What about the warehouse or places these items were stored before being placed on display? Many warehouses contain insects or rodents of some sort, to which these items may have been exposed. Shoppers should always wear something to protect their skin when trying on clothes, or simply wait until you get home and wash it.

Video consoles, computers, phones, and televisions—think about how many stores have these on display for customers to try out while deciding whether to make the purchase. I am almost certain that none of these devices are ever cleaned after customers have been touching them. Although bacteria can oftentimes live on the skin without causing an infection, the risk of getting a bacterial skin infection becomes higher when the skin is broken. There are many different types of bacterial infections that can penetrate through the skin, but there are a few that are more frequent than others. Let's use our common sense and start cleaning and sanitizing our items.

IF YOU DIDN'T KNOW, NOW YOU KNOW!

HOUSEKEEPERS

Housekeepers are typically a luxury for those of us who do not have time to spare in cleaning our homes ourselves but want to ensure that things look clean and organized. We almost never think about the supplies, products, or equipment that our housekeepers may be using in our home or if they're harboring someone else's germs. Let me elaborate on that a little more. Typically housekeepers have more than one client, and they usually use their own items to clean with. Well, what happens when they've used their vacuum cleaner at a home that has a pet with a flea infestation or, better yet, a room full of bedbugs? The same vacuum cleaner is then used at your home, being a transporter of germs or heaven knows what else. At best they should be using your vacuum cleaner. How clean are the cleaning products they're using? Let me explain. Usually they're using gloves, but they have to touch the apparatus that the cleaning product is in. Are they changing their gloves in between each spray and wipe? I'm almost certain the answer is no. I doubt if every housekeeper is purchasing new cleaning products or wipes for each home they clean. What surfaces are these items being placed on when not in use (bathroom floor, countertop, bathtub, etc.)? Let's look at it this way: Every home has its own type of germs posing as invited guests. Why would you want to invite someone else's germs into your home? It is best to have your housekeeper use your products that are in your home.

MAIL

Almost everyone gets mail on a regular basis. If not, then you're one of the lucky few. Let's think about the process of sending a letter via mail. The letter is usually placed in an envelope or package by a person who either seals it by licking it or applying some other type of sealant. Once the letter arrives at the post office, it then goes through a sorting process and is touched by several more hands. By the time your mail arrives to your home, it's unknown exactly how many hands have touched it or if it was sealed with spit! With this being known, wouldn't it make common sense to wash your hands after opening your mail?

MALLS

There are not too many people I know who do not like going to the mall, even if it's just to window shop or simply to get out and get a little exercise. Either way, the mall is a melting pot for germs. Hundreds of people crowd into malls regularly, touching and trying on things, but how often are those things cleaned? Most stores have samples on display such as creams, lotions, perfumes, etc., which is a free-for-all, but who wants to use these items after everyone has touched and tried them on? A new spray bottle or a sample is not placed on display daily; it typically stays out until it's empty. How many people do you think in a typical day use these sample items? It would be wise to wash your hands after handling sample items.

MONEY

Money transactions are conducted every day. People are constantly handling and handing money from person to person, machine, or device. We use our debit cards regularly and without any thought, we return them to their original place in our purse or wallet. I feel that it would be common sense to not only wash your hands after handling money and coins but to also clean your debit/credit card after using it. Again, germs tend to harbor in dark, cool places. A wallet or a purse would be a great place to hide if I were a germ.

NAIL SALONS

Initially when you walk into a nail salon, the first question asked is, "What are you getting?" And depending on your response, the employee usually proceeds to start on your pedicure/manicure. I have never seen any employees at nail shops I have visited wash their hands before working with a client. It's not certain how or if their files, buffers, etc., are cleaned between clients. I dare not imagine how many germs have collected on these items. I usually see the employees rushing between clients, trying to get them in and out, tending to their children, eating, waxing eyebrows, and handling money. None of these tasks are out of the "norm," but it would be exceptional if at least on one of my visits, I observed an employee washing their hands. A simple solution to decrease the risk of spreading germs or a potential infection if your skin is accidently broken would be to ask them to use new files or take your own items in with you. This will protect you and potentially other customers from the spread of germs.

OFFICE

There usually is an abundance of pens or computers in most office settings. Often, employees may grab a pen off of their coworker's desk or even log in to their computer without giving thought to what their coworker may have done with that pen or keyboard. A great deal of people subconsciously tend to chew on the ends of their pen/pencils or eat at their desks during breaks without giving thought to who may have touched that ink pen/pencil or keyboard before them. Some people work through lunch, therefore touching food, then touching the keyboard, and possibly licking a finger or two in between. For those of you who feel some sense of gratification when you swipe a "good writing" pen, ask yourself how many other people have used that pen.

RESTAURANTS

We live in a "microwave age," some would say, as we pack our restaurants every day while attempting to avoid the hustle and bustle of preparing a meal at home. I for one was not a big fan of cooking every day and enjoyed an occasional meal out of the home until I realized how many unnecessary germs I was exposing myself to. The restaurant routine always started the same way. Upon entering the establishment with my family, I would be greeted by a server, who would grab the menus, utensils, plates, etc. (depending on the restaurant), before showing us to our seats. The first thing that comes to mind is the thought of how many other people have touched the menu and if they ever clean them. Take a moment to remember the times you have gone out to eat and had to practically pull the menu apart with both hands because it was stuck together from some sort of guck. Then the next thought that comes to mind is about the server and how long it had been since the last time he/she washed their hands.

The worse part of my restaurant experience is when I receive unclean silverware. It should only take a moment for the person who is wrapping or placing the silverware on the table to notice food particles. I understand that dishwashers may break, staff is limited, or whatever the circumstance may be, but it is too great of a health risk not to ensure that your silverware is clean before placing it on tables. I for one prefer to use plastic utensils that are individually wrapped to cut down on the risk of the spread of germs. Notice how most buffets have the plates already sitting on the buffet line and the silverware is in a basket or container, free for everyone to touch. I've watched people pick up a plate or piece of silverware that was not clean and simply place it to the side or back in its original place, then the next unassuming person gets the luck of the draw. I shun thinking about how unclean the hands of some of those people were.

I was once laughed at for using a straw and plastic silverware in an upscale restaurant, but when you've experienced lipstick stains on your glass and food on your silverware, it gives things a new perspective. Safety from the prevention of the spread of germs is not laughable but plausible for me.

SHOES

We walk around all day wearing the same shoes, traveling from place to place, collecting all types of stuff on the soles. If it's easy for a rock to get stuck in the groove of the sole of a shoe, imagine how easy it is for a germ to cling to it.

After wearing your shoes during the day, you should take into consideration that they are soiled, and why would you want to walk around in your home with soiled shoes? I suggest taking your shoes off at the door to decrease the spread of germs in your home. Many of us have small children or pets that spend most of their time playing on the floor. It increases their susceptibility to germs and infections when you walk across your carpet, hardwood, or tiled floors.

SHOE SHOPPERS

I love shoe shopping, and there is actually an art to "safe" shoe shopping. The cardinal rule in shopping for shoes is to never try them on with your bare feet. You should bring your own socks. I also avoid using the stockinet or socks that the store provides because there is potential that other customers could have worn them before they were offered to you. As I mentioned in previous chapters, items are stored and shipped from warehouses, where they have possibly been exposed to unfavorable environments, rodents, etc. Then once shipped, the items undergo handling by multiple people. You have to consider the cleanliness of other customers when trying on shoes. Are there any open wounds on their feet? Do they have athlete's foot or some other type of fungus? Shoes should be cleaned prior to wearing them. Again, not only have these items been sitting in a warehouse before being shipped, I doubt if the salesperson is washing their hands between helping people try on shoes, handling the money, and restocking merchandise.

LAUNDROMATS

People need to be aware of the potential spread of germs when taking their clothes to a Laundromat. Clothes are being brought in every day from different types of environments, then transferred from washer to dryer without any sanitizing between each use. It is seldom that an attendant is present in these settings. Newer front-loader washers have sanitizing mechanisms installed, but what about the older washers that still have buildup along the insides of the machine and in the dispenser cups? The thought is that washers are automatically cleaned, but they are not. If you clean out your car or your refrigerator, why not clean your washer/dryer? It gets as equally dirty.

EXPECTANT MOTHERS

Moms, please stop letting everyone touch your baby bumps, especially strangers! It is second nature to want to rub a pregnant belly when you see one, but not only is it invasive, it's unsanitary if your hands are not clean. Most moms-to-be do not want to appear rude, but they need to think about the possible health risk they're placing themselves in, and maybe then they may not have an issue with placing a stop to the occasional belly rubs.

TIPS AND TECHNIQUES

Library – use an antibacterial/disinfectant wipe or spray when checking out books at the library, you can bet that several people have touched the same book before you did.

Movies, public transportation – think about the many different people that have sat in the seat before you, it would be beneficial to use an antibacterial disinfectant spray before sitting in that seat.

Tolls – ask yourself, "why does the attendant wear gloves?" Since it's impossible to wash your hands while driving, you should always have an antibacterial hand sanitizer available.

Toys – always disinfect before and after your child and his/her friends finishing playing with them

www.ingramcontent.com/pod-product-compliance
Lightning Source LLC
Chambersburg PA
CBHW061521180526
45171CB00001B/283